KETO VEGETARIAN DIET: *A Vegetarian Approach To Burn Fat, Be Mindful And Beat Inflammation*

RACHEL RUSH

CONTENTS

Legal and Disclaimer

The information contained in this book is not designed to replace or take the place of any form of medicine or professional medical advice. The information in this book has been provided for educational and entertainment purposes only.

The information contained in this book has been compiled from sources deemed reliable, and it is accurate to the best of the Author's knowledge; however, the Author cannot guarantee its accuracy and validity and cannot be held liable for any omissions or errors. Changes are periodically made to this book. You must consult your doctor or get professional medical advice before using any of the suggested remedies, techniques, or information in this book. Upon using the information contained in this book, you agree to hold harmless the Author from and against any damages, costs, and expenses, including any legal fees potentially resulting from the application of any of the information provided by this book. This disclaimer applies to any damages or injury caused by the use and application, whether directly or indirectly, of any advice or information presented, whether for breach of contract, tort, negligence, personal injury, criminal intent, or under any other cause of action.

You agree to accept all risks of using the information presented inside this book. Consult a professional medical practitioner to ensure you are both able and healthy enough to partecipate.

Vegetarian or Vegetarian?

Are you a vegetarian or a vegetarian? The distinction between these two dietary lifestyle choices might seem slight, but these two options have very different implications for eating choices and nutrition. Vegetarians choose not to eat meat: mammal, fish or poultry. However, vegetarians do not exclude products which are animal derivatives, such as eggs, milk, and cheeses.

Vegetarians, on the other hand, do not eat anything of animal origin. They choose a strictly vegetarian diet consuming only foods which are of plant origin. They do not consume eggs, milk, cheeses or any derivatives or foods that contain these derivatives. Vegetarians are, in other words, people who choose not to use any product which is made from the exploitation of animals. For this reason, they also do not wear leather, silk, or fur, nor do they use cosmetics tested on animals, or participate in sports where animals are involved.

We can conclude that while neither vegetarians nor vegetarians eat meat, the term vegetarian indicates a dietary choice, and the word vegetarian signifies a comprehensive lifestyle choice.

Keto for Vegetarians and Vegetarians

Can vegetarians follow a keto diet? They absolutely can! If you've given up meat for ethical or health reasons but you're interested in lowering your carb intake, Keto is for you.

Are there health concerns? There could be some mineral and nutrient deficiencies, but this would depend on how restricted your diet is.

Keto can be used in most vegetarian dietary regimes, however the "vegetarian" as opposed to "vegetarian" diet will allow for more meal choices. Humans need to consume protein, which contains all nine essential amino acids. While animal protein contains all nine, plants do not.

Vegetarians will employ a combination of legumes, seeds, and grains to get those necessary amino acids. But many of these foods are high in carbs and cannot be used in a keto lifestyle. In order to achieve ketosis, you will need to limit your carbs per day.

If you consume keto low carb protein from plants such as seeds or nuts, you will be able to satisfy your body's nutrition requirements. Hemp seeds, for example, are a great provider of protein for vegetarians and vegetarians alike. Vegetarians will not have any problems with the keto lifestyle because they can consume dairy and will be able to satisfy any nutrition concerns.

With attentive planning, vegetarians can also benefit from the keto lifestyle. They can utilize high-fat products, which are plant-based, such as avocados, nuts, seeds, and even coconut oil. Vegetarian diets, like Keto diets, are linked to weight loss, prevention of heart disease, and diabetes. So, whether you're a vegetarian or a vegetarian, stock up on coconut products, nuts and seeds, tofu, non-starchy vegetables, avocados, and avocado and olive oils, and enjoy all the benefits that a Keto vegetarian or Keto vegetarian way of life has to offer.

BREAKFAST

Tomato and Asparagus Frittata

If you enjoy eggs for breakfast, this tasty Italian omelet will help you get your day off to a great start. It's nutritious and easy to make, and best of all, it's a low-carb Keto dish.

- 10-minute prep time
- Cooking time: 20 minutes
- 6 servings

Nutritional Information:

Carbohydrates: 14.3 g
Fat: 9.6 g
Protein: 8.9 g
Calories: 168

What you need:

- 250 grams of trimmed, fresh asparagus
- 4 small onions, cleaned and sliced
- 6 eggs
- 10 cherry tomatoes
- 2 tablespoons of extra virgin olive oil
- 4 tablespoons of Parmesan cheese, freshly grated
- Salt and ground black pepper to taste

What to do:

- Fill a medium-sized pot with water and bring it to a boil. Cook your asparagus in the boiling water for approximately 10 minutes or until the asparagus is tender.
- Preheat the broiler setting in your oven.

- Now heat the olive oil in your favorite frying pan and then add the onions, cherry tomatoes and asparagus. Cook for 1 to 2 minutes.
- In a bowl, beat the eggs well and add salt and pepper to taste. Add in the grated Parmesan cheese and blend it together well with the eggs.
- Finally, add the egg and cheese mixture into your frying pan and cook for 7 to 8 minutes. The bottom of your frittata should be firm, and the top should be almost set.
- Place the frittata under your broiler for another 3 minutes or until the top is firm and slightly browned.

Slide your frittata onto a serving platter, cut and serve.

Artichoke and Spinach Egg Casserole

Looking for something scrumptious but keto-friendly for a special breakfast or brunch? Look no further. This delightful egg casserole is rich in taste and low on carbs.

- Prep Time: 15 minutes
- Cooking time: 35 minutes
- Serves 10 to 12

Nutritional Information:

Carbohydrates: 3.3 g
Fat: 8.5 g
Protein: 11.9 g
Calories: 141

What you need:

- 16 eggs
- 14 ounces of artichoke hearts
- 10 ounces of spinach
- ¼ cup of almond milk
- ½ cup of freshly grated Parmesan cheese
- ½ cup of ricotta cheese
- 1 cup of cheddar cheese, shredded
- ¼ cup of diced onion
- 1 clove of garlic, finely minced
- 1 teaspoon of your preferred salt
- ½ of a teaspoon of dried thyme
- ½ of a teaspoon of ground red pepper

What to do:

- Turn on your oven and preheat it at 350 degrees Fahrenheit. With nonstick cooking spray, spray a rectangular baking dish of 9 x 13 inches.
- Crack your eggs into a bowl and add in the almond milk. Whisk the eggs and milk until blended well.
- Cut your artichoke hearts into small pieces and separate all the leaves. Remove any excess water from your spinach by squeezing in paper towels. Once completed, add both the artichokes and the spinach to you egg and milk mixture. Now add in the shredded cheddar cheese, the grated Parmesan cheese, the diced onion, the minced garlic, thyme, salt and red pepper to the egg mixture. Blend together all the ingredients and pour the mixture into the prepared baking pan.
- Place dollops of ricotta cheese evenly on top of the entire egg mixture. It should be spread completely on all of the egg mixture.
- Place in your preheated oven for about 35 minutes until completely cooked. The egg casserole should not jiggle when you move the pan.

Serve family and guests this great breakfast choice.

Parmesan Asparagus with Baked Eggs

Want a quick, satisfying breakfast that's tasty and low-carb? If you like baked eggs or are an asparagus fan, this tempting breakfast entrée will make your day.

- Prep Time: 10 minutes (with room temperature eggs)
- Cooking time: 18 minutes
- Serves: 2

Nutritional Information:

Carbohydrates: 4.4 g
Fat: 13.8 g
Protein: 13.5 g
Calories: 188

What you need:

- 8 good sized asparagus spears
- 4 eggs at room temperature
- 2 tablespoons of freshly grated Parmesan cheese
- 2 tablespoons of extra virgin olive oil
- Salt to taste
- Freshly ground black pepper to taste

What to do:

- Turn on your oven and preheat it to 400 degrees Fahrenheit (200° Celsius). Grease two gratin dishes with olive oil.
- Crack the four eggs into 4 separate small dishes and allow them to reach room temperature before using.

- Take your 8 asparagus spears and slice off the tougher stem part at the bottom. Now cut each spear into diagonally shaped short pieces.
- Place half of your asparagus pieces equally into the two individual gratin dishes and roast your asparagus for 10 minutes (setting a timer).
- When the timer rings, take one of the asparagus dishes from the oven and place two room temperature eggs over the asparagus. Now place the asparagus and eggs back into the oven and set your timer for another five minutes. Do this with the second gratin dish as well.
- When the timer rings, remove the gratin dishes and sprinkle a tablespoon of the freshly grated Parmesan on each gratin dish. Place the dishes back in the oven and cook for another three minutes. The egg white should be set, and the cheese melted.

Serve this appetizing breakfast entrée hot allowing the egg yolk to run freely over the asparagus.

Green Keto Smoothie

No time for breakfast because you're on the go? Try this keto super food smoothie. It's high in fiber and low in carbs and will help you start your day energized and focused. It takes all of 5 minutes to prepare and is great tasting.

- Prep Time: 5 minutes
- Cooking time: 0 minutes
- Serves: 1

Nutritional Information:

Carbohydrates: 19.8 g
Fat: 62.5 g
Protein: 10.7 g
Calories: 627

What you need:

- 2/3 packed cup of fresh spinach
- ½ of a medium ripe avocado
- 1 tablespoon of MCT oil *
- 1 teaspoon of vanilla extract
- ½ teaspoon of matcha powder **
- ½ cup of almond milk or coconut milk
- ¼ cup of vegetarian protein powder
- 1 tablespoon of monk fruit sweetener
- 2/3 cup of water
- 5 to 6 ice cubes

**MCT oil or Medium-chain triglycerides are a kind of fat usually extracted from coconut or palm kernel oils. It is an outstanding* *source of good fats. It can be purchased at your local health food store or on line.*

*** Matcha powder is made from stone grounding green tea leaves.*

What to do:

Place all of your ingredients into your blender and blend on high until smooth. You can add additional water depending on how thick you like your smoothie.

Now take on the day!

Breakfast Mushroom and spinach casserole

This light, keto vegetarian breakfast casserole will leave your family asking for second helpings. This delicious breakfast dish will satiate you and satisfy your taste buds as well. This is a great way to begin your day or a fantastic addition to a vegetarian brunch.

- Prep Time: 15 minutes
- Cooking time: 45 minutes
- Serves: 8

Nutritional Information:

Carbohydrates: 7.4 g
Fat: 25.9 g
Protein: 25 g
Calories: 358

What you need:

- 6 beaten eggs
- One 12-ounce bag of fresh spinach
- 3 sliced green onions
- 1 chopped medium yellow or white onion
- ½ lb. of sliced fresh mushrooms
- 2 minced garlic cloves
- 5 tablespoons of unsalted butter
- 16 ounces of cottage cheese
- 12 ounces of freshly grated sharp cheddar cheese
- 1 teaspoon of salt
- ½ of a teaspoon of freshly ground black pepper

What to do:

- Turn on your oven to 350 degrees Fahrenheit. Use one tablespoon of unsalted butter to grease a 9 x 13-inch baking pan or dish.
- Heat the remaining four tablespoons of butter in your favorite skillet and sauté the onions, garlic and mushrooms for 4 to 5 minutes until the onions are soft and translucent and the mushrooms are soft.
- Now add the spinach gradually into the skillet and sauté. Cover your skillet and allow the spinach to wilt. This should take another 4 to 5 minutes.
- Let the mixture cool. Drain any excess liquid.
- In a medium-sized bowl, whisk together the eggs, cottage and cheddar cheeses and the salt and pepper to taste.
- Add the mushroom and spinach into the egg and cheese mixture.
- Stir gently, blending well and pour the mixture into your baking dish.
- Bake for 45 to50 minutes making sure that the center of the casserole is cooked and that the casserole has a nice golden-brown top.

Enjoy, enjoy, enjoy!

Tunisian Keto Shakshuka

This is a wonderful breakfast entrée from Tunisia but is common throughout the Middle East. It is an appetizing twist on poached eggs, which are bathed in a tomato and chili pepper sauce. So, if you want to try something other than scrambled eggs or once over easy, this tantalizing dish will give you one more reason to look forward to breakfast.

- Prep Time: 10 minutes
- Cooking time: 10 minutes
- Serves: 1

What you need:

- 4 eggs
- 1 chili pepper
- 1 cup of tomato or marinara sauce
- 1 ounce of Greek feta cheese
- 1/8 teaspoon of cumin
- fresh basil, chopped
- salt to taste
- freshly ground black pepper to taste

What to do:

- Turn on your oven and preheat it to 400 degrees Fahrenheit (200° Celsius).
- Take a small-sized frying pan or skillet and heat the marinara or tomato sauce and the chili pepper over a medium flame. Cook the chili pepper for at least 5 minutes.
- Remove the skillet from the flame.
- Now crack your eggs and place them in the sauce.

- Sprinkle crumbled feta cheese onto your eggs and the cumin for seasoning.
- Add salt and freshly ground black pepper to taste.
- Place the heated skillet with your ingredients into your oven and bake for 10 minutes.
- When the eggs have been cooked (yokes should be runny), remove the skillet from the oven and serve with freshly chopped basil as a topping.

Cauliflower Hash Browns with Scrambled Vegetarian Eggs

Cauliflower is a great source of minerals and vitamins, but it's also a wonderful substitute for those addicting starches that we love to accompany our meals with. So, if you can't imagine living without a portion of hash brown potatoes at breakfast, or at any other meal for that matter, try cauliflower hash browns. This delicious vegetable substitute will change your opinion and your waistline!

For the hash browns:

- Prep Time: 5 to 10 minutes
- Cooking time: 10 to 15 minutes
- Serves: 5 to 6

What you need:

- 1 head of cauliflower cut into small florets
- 2 tablespoons of coconut oil
- 1 chopped onion
- 1 teaspoon of garlic powder
- ½ cup of chickpea flour
- 2 tablespoons of cornstarch
- 1 teaspoon of salt
- 2 tablespoons of water

What to do:

- Turn on your oven and preheat it to 400 degrees Fahrenheit (200° Celsius). Spray your baking sheet with oil and set aside.
- Using your food processor or a box grater, grate the cauliflower and onion into small crumbly rice-like pieces.

- Now, in a bowl, add the chickpea flour, garlic powder, corn starch, salt and water to the cauliflower and onions and blend completely.
- Separate your mixture into 10 to 12 separate portions and form your hash brown patties.
- Place your patties onto your baking sheet and bake for 40 minutes, flipping them to the other side after 20 minutes. If you're in a hurry, you can heat the patties in a skillet with some coconut oil, cooking for 5 minutes on each side.

For your Vegetarian Scrambled Eggs:

What you need:

- 1 14-ounce package of tofu
- 3 tablespoons of avocado oil
- 2 tablespoons of finely diced white or yellow onion
- 1 cup of fresh baby spinach
- 3 cherry tomatoes, diced
- ½ teaspoon of garlic powder
- ½ teaspoon of salt
- ½ teaspoon of turmeric
- 3 ounces of vegetarian cheddar cheese

What to do:

- Dry your tofu block with paper towels, squeezing out gently any excess water.
- In a frying pan, over medium heat, sauté the finely diced onion in 1/3 of the avocado oil. The onion should be translucent and soft.
- Now place your block of tofu into the skillet and mash it with a fork until it has the appearance of scrambled eggs.
- Sprinkle with the remaining oil, garlic powder, turmeric and salt and toss gently to blend in the seasonings.

- Cook your tofu on medium heat, stirring gently until the liquid has evaporated.
- Now fold in your baby spinach, the diced cherry tomatoes and the vegetarian cheddar cooking for another two minutes. The cheese should melt, and the spinach should wilt.
- Serve hot with your cauliflower hash brown patties!

Keto Brownie Muffins

If you think of brownies, you certainly don't think diet. And nothing about a brownie or a muffin suggests keto. Well surprise! You can have these delicious brownie muffins without violating your keto way of life. Chocolaty and sweet, this keto recipe will start your day off with a real boost to your energy.

- Prep Time: 15 minutes
- Cooking time: 20 minutes
- Serves: 8

What you need:

- 6 tablespoons of melted coconut oil
- 1 teaspoon of vanilla extract
- 3 large eggs
- ¼ cup of coconut cream
- 1 cup of almond flour
- 2 tablespoons of almond milk
- 2 teaspoons of baking powder
- ½ cup of erythritol
- stevia to taste
- ½ cup of unsweetened cacao powder
- 3 tablespoons of ground chia seeds
- ½ cup of chopped walnuts

What to do:

- Turn on your oven and preheat it to 350 degrees Fahrenheit (175° Celsius).
- Take the 6 tablespoons of coconut oil and place them in a microwave safe dish. Now met your coconut oil using your

microwave for intervals of 10 seconds until melted. Set aside to cool.

- In a bowl, combine the eggs, vanilla extract, almond milk and coconut cream and whisk them thoroughly.
- In another bowl, mix together the baking powder, almond flour, erythritol, cacao powder and the ground chia seeds. (You can use a blender to ground your chia seeds.) You may wish to add some stevia if you want them to be a little sweeter. Finally stir in the chopped walnuts. The walnuts should be chopped into very small pieces.
- When the coconut oil has cooled sufficiently, it should be whisked into the egg mixture. Stir well. Now add the egg mixture to the almond flour and cacao powder mixture. Blend really well.
- Divide your batter into 6 equal parts and place them in a muffin tray that has been greased or alternatively, use cupcake paper baking cups.
- Place in the oven and bake for approximately 20 minutes. You may wish to insert a cake tester to judge if they are baked through.
- Set your brownie muffins aside to cool. Before removing them, run a knife around the brownie. Enjoy!

Keto Coffee Cake

Everybody loves a piece of freshly baked coffee cake. And who says a diet is synonymous with deprivation? Who says you can't have your cake and eat it too? Guess what? With a keto life style, you can eat coffee cake. This scrumptious cinnamon coffee cake will make you happy you're following a keto lifestyle and will delight any non-keto followers who taste it as well.

- Prep Time: 10 minutes
- Cooking time: 45 to 50 minutes
- Serves 10

What you need for the coffee cake:

- 2 eggs
- 1 cup of sour cream
- ½ cup of cooled melted butter
- 2 cups of almond flour
- 2 teaspoons of baking powder
- 1 ¼ cup of sugar substitute
- ¼ teaspoon of nutmeg
- 2 ½ teaspoons of cinnamon
- ¼ teaspoon of baking soda
- 1 teaspoon of salt

What you need for the cake topping:

- ½ cup of almond flour
- ¼ cup of sugar substitute
- ¼ cup of coconut flour
- ¼ cup of chopped pecans
- 1 teaspoon of cinnamon

- ¼ cup of thinly sliced cold butter
- 1/8 teaspoon of salt

What to do:

- Turn on your oven and preheat it to 350 degrees Fahrenheit (175° Celsius).
- Grease a 9-inch sized spring-form or push pan cake pan with butter.
- In a small bowl, prepare your topping. Combine the almond flour, coconut flour, sugar substitute, cinnamon, chopped pecans and salt. Now add the thinly sliced butter pieces and mix together with the dry ingredients until you achieve a crumbly mixture. Set it aside.
- In a rather large mixing bowl, prepare your cake batter. Mix together the almond flour, baking powder, sugar substitute, nutmeg, cinnamon, baking soda, and sea salt.
- In a separate smaller bowl, blend the melted butter, sour cream and the eggs together thoroughly. Now add the butter mixture into the dry mixture. Stir until well blended.
- Place the batter into your cake pan. Sprinkle the topping you prepared, completely over the top of the cake batter.
- Place in the oven and bake your coffee cake for at least 45 to 50 minutes. The crumble topping should be slightly browned. A cake tester or toothpick should come out clean after poking your cake if it is completely baked.
- Allow your coffee cake to cool before slicing and serving.

Keto Vegetarian Porridge

If you love hot cereals, this keto porridge will keep you feeling satiated right up to lunchtime. It's easy to fix and can be customized to your preferred flavors. Creamy and thick, you'll need only a few minutes to prepare this tasty breakfast alternative.

- Prep Time: 5 minutes
- Cooking time: 5 minutes
- Serves: 1

What you need:

- 3 tablespoons of flaxseed meal
- 2 tablespoons of coconut flour
- 1 ½ cups of almond milk which is unsweetened
- 2 tablespoons of vegetarian protein powder*
- erythritol to taste

*You can find vegetarian protein powder in various flavors. Choose your favorite!

What to do:

1. Combine the flaxseed meal, coconut flour and protein powder in a bowl, mixing well.
2. Place the mixture in a saucepan and add the almond milk. Cook at medium heat.
3. As it thickens you should mix in your sweetener to taste. If you're making this cereal for the first time, try adding approximately ½ tablespoon of sweetener to begin with.

4. Serve with your preferred toppings. Possible toppings include blueberries, peaches, blackberries, raspberries, strawberries, cinnamon, or even unsweetened coconut.

APPETIZERS

Spinach and Avocado Dip

Having a party and looking for that perfect smooth and creamy vegetarian dip to serve that won't interfere with your keto life style? This dip is the creamiest non-dairy appetizer you can serve, and you don't have to be a vegetarian or keto follower to enjoy it.

- Prep Time: 15 minutes
- Cooking time: 0 minutes
- Serves: 12

What you need:

- ½ cup of spinach (about 20 large leaves of spinach) that has been blanched in boiling water for 2 to 3 minutes. Then squeezed and drained.
- 1 crushed garlic clove
- 2 large avocados that are ripe. This should produce about 2 cups of mashed avocado.
- ¼ cup of chopped fresh coriander*
- ¾ cup of dairy free yogurt
- 4 tablespoons of extra virgin avocado oil**
- 1 tablespoon of lime juice
- ½ teaspoon of salt
- Freshly ground black pepper to taste

**Coriander or cilantro can be substituted with your favorite fresh herb such as basil, mint or parsley.*
***Avocado oil can be substituted with extra virgin olive oil.*

What to do:

- Trim your spinach leaves and put them in a large bowl. Cover the spinach with boiling water. Cover the bowl and set aside.

- After 2 to 3 minutes, drain the spinach and rinse with cold water. Now squeeze the spinach leaves to eliminate any excess water and pat the spinach dry with paper towels.
- In a blender or food processor, combine the spinach, the mashed ripe avocado, crushed garlic, yogurt, coriander, lime juice, 3 tablespoons of avocado oil and salt and pepper.
- Blend on high for 2 to 3 minutes until smooth.
- Pour into a serving bowl. Drizzle the remaining tablespoon of avocado oil on the top.
- Place in the refrigerator for at least 30 minutes before serving.

Serve with your favorite dippers.

Caprese Eggplant Roll Ups

Great flavor from fresh vegetables wed with delicious cheese make for a delightful appetizer to begin your dinner with.

- Prep Time: 5 minutes
- Cooking time: 8 minutes
- Serves: 8

What you need:

- 1 medium Aubergine eggplant
- 4 ounces of mozzarella cheese
- 1 large tomato
- 2 to 6 fresh basil leaves
- extra virgin olive oil

What to do:

- Cut the ends off of your eggplant. Now cut the eggplant into thin slices lengthwise. Remove any small slices or skin pieces and discard.
- Slice both the tomato and the mozzarella into thin slices.
- Shred the fresh basil leaves into thin pieces.
- Warm your griddle pan over medium heat. Brush the olive oil on the eggplant slices. Now grill the eggplant slices for several minutes on both sides.
- When the second side is almost grilled, place a piece of mozzarella cheese onto the larger thicker part of the eggplant slice. Now top the mozzarella with a piece of tomato. Place a smaller piece of mozzarella onto the smaller end of the eggplant slice. Add on some shredded basil, drizzle some olive oil and grind some fresh black pepper on top.

- Cook for another minute or so and then transfer from your griddle pan to a dish carefully. Allow for any excess juices to drain off.
- Roll your eggplant starting with the smaller, thinner end. Once it has closed, fasten it with a toothpick or cocktail stick. Serve warm.

Serve with your favorite dippers.

Broccoli and Cheese Fritters with Sauce

If you're not a broccoli fan, you could very well become one after tasting these tantalizing fritter appetizers. Crunchy on the outside with a soft inside, they taste absolutely delicious.

- Prep Time: 10 minutes
- Cooking time: 5 minutes
- Yields 16 fritters

What you need:

- 4 ounces of fresh broccoli
- 4 ounces of mozzarella cheese
- ¾ cup of almond flour
- 2 large eggs
- ¼ cup plus 3 tablespoons of flaxseed meal
- 2 teaspoons of baking powder
- salt and freshly ground black pepper to taste

For your sauce:

- ¼ cup of mayonnaise
- ¼ of fresh dill, chopped
- ½ tablespoon of lemon juice
- salt and freshly ground pepper to taste

What to do:

- Place your broccoli into a food processor or blender and process/blend until reduced to rice sized pieces

- In a mixing bowl, combine the almond flour, cheese, ¼ cup of flaxseed meal, the baking powder and the broccoli. Add your salt and freshly ground black pepper to taste.
- Now add in the eggs and stir until everything is well blended.
- Roll your batter into 16 balls. Coat the balls with the three tablespoons of flaxseed meal.
- Heat a deep fat fryer to 375 Fahrenheit and lay the fritters into the frying basket. Do not overfill the basket.
- Fry your fritters for about three to five minutes until golden. Place the fritters on paper towels to absorb any excess grease.
- Blend the mayonnaise, dill and lemon juice for your sauce. Season to taste. Now serve your fritters and enjoy.

Cauliflower Hummus

Love the traditional chickpea hummus but you want low carbs? Try this appetizing cauliflower hummus. You'll be hard-pressed to tell the difference. This hummus is egg free, gluten free, grain free, nut free and dairy free. Wow!

- Prep Time: 10 minutes
- Cooking time: 15 minutes
- Yields: Six servings (¼ cup each)

What you need:

- 3 cups of raw cauliflower florets
- 5 tablespoons of extra virgin olive oil
- 2 tablespoons of water
- 3 garlic cloves, whole
- 2 raw crushed garlic cloves
- 1 ½ tablespoons of Tahini paste
- ½ teaspoon of salt
- ¾ teaspoon of salt
- 3 tablespoons of lemon juice
- smoked paprika
- extra virgin olive oil for serving

What to do:

- Place the cauliflower, water, 2 tablespoons of extra virgin olive oil, ½ teaspoon of salt and three whole garlic cloves into a microwave safe dish and mix gently. Cook in the microwave for about fifteen minutes until softened and darkened in color.
- Place the cauliflower mixture into your blender or food processor and blend well. Now ad in the Tahini paste, lemon

juice, 2 raw crushed garlic cloves, 3 tablespoons of extra virgin olive oil and ¾ teaspoon of salt. Blend thoroughly until smooth in texture. Adjust the seasoning to taste.

- Place your hummus mixture in a bowl and sprinkle on some extra virgin olive oil and some smoked paprika. Now serve with celery sticks, tart apple slices, chips of raw radish or your favorite dippers.

Cheesy Hearts of Palm Dip

Missing those gooey cheesy hot dips? This wonderful dip uses the vegetable "hearts of palm" that is low carb. This is the core of various types of palm trees. It is high in fiber, zinc, iron potassium and various minerals making this dip super healthy as well as yummy.

- Prep Time: 15 minutes
- Cooking time: 20 to 25 minutes
- Yields: Six servings (3 tablespoons each)

What you need:

- 1 14 ounce can, drained, of hearts of palms
- ¼ cup of mayonnaise
- 3 stalks of chopped green onions
- 2 tablespoons of Italian seasoning
- 2 large eggs (Separate the yoke from the white in one of the eggs.)
- ½ cup of shredded fresh Parmesan cheese
- ¼ cup of freshly grated Parmesan cheese for the topping

What to do:

- Heat your oven to 350 degrees Fahrenheit (175° Celsius) and spray a small baking dish with nonstick cooking spray.
- Chop up the bulbs of your green onions and rain the can of hearts of palms.
- Place the hearts of palms, Parmesan cheese, onion, seasoning and mayonnaise into your food processor or blender. Pulse until the mixture is chopped up well.

- Now add one whole egg plus one egg yolk into the blender/food processor. Pulse three to four times to mix the ingredients.
- Now pour your mixture into the baking dish you prepared and cook for 15 to 20 minutes until the mixture puffs up. Stir it and a more Parmesan cheese on top.
- Now broil your dip until the top melts and begins to brown.
- Serve hot with your favorite vegetarian dippers.

Keto Ranch Dip

If you love Ranch dressing, this tangy version of the dip goes great with snacks, salads or veggies. Make this terrific fresh dip of your own and you'll never buy a bottle at the store again.

- Prep Time: 5 minutes
- Chill time: 20 minutes
- Yields: 8 servings

What you need:

- 1 cup mayonnaise
- ½ cup sour cream
- 2 tablespoons ranch seasoning*

**Make your own ranch seasoning by mixing together 2 tablespoons of dried chives, 2 tablespoons of parsley flakes, 2 tablespoons of dill flakes, 1 tablespoon of powdered garlic, 1 tablespoon of powdered onion, 1 tablespoon salt, and ½ tablespoon black pepper. Place in an airtight jar or container.*

What to do:

Blend the ingredients together in a medium-sized bowl and refrigerate for at least 15 to 20 minutes to allow the flavors to amalgamate.

Serve your dip with your favorite veggies or dippers.

Keto Tzatziki

This is a very low carb version of the traditional Greek dip Tzatziki.

- Prep Time: 10 minutes
- Chill time: 20 minutes
- Yields: 4 servings

What you need:

- 1 cucumber
- 5.3 ounces of plain Greek yogurt (150 grams)
- 2 teaspoons of garlic paste
- 1 tablespoon of fresh dill, chopped
- 2 teaspoons of lemon juice
- Salt
- Freshly ground black pepper

What to do:

- Slice your cucumber across the middle. Now divide each half into 4 quarters lengthwise. Remove the strip of cucumber seeds in the middle. Discard. Grate or chop finely the cucumber remaining.
- Mix into the cucumber, the Greek yogurt, lemon juice, garlic, and fresh chopped dill. Stir blending well. Add salt and pepper to taste.
- Refrigerate and serve with your favorite vegetables or dippers.

Serve your dip with your favorite veggies or dippers.

Keto Cream Cheese with Herbs

This is a popular tangy dip to serve as an appetizer. It takes very little time to prepare and can be served with the vegetables or dippers of your choosing. It's a traditional favorite and very low carb. A popular dip for vegetarians and non-vegetarians alike.

- Prep Time: 5 minutes
- Chill time: 20 minutes
- Yields: 8 servings

What you need:

- 8 ounces of softened cream cheese
- 1 tablespoon of fresh or dried dill
- 1 tablespoon of fresh or dried chives
- 3 finely minced garlic cloves*
- 1 teaspoon of extra virgin olive oil
- Salt to taste
- Freshly ground black pepper to taste
- Celery stalks

What to do:

- Stir the ingredients into your cream cheese. Now refrigerate for at least fifteen minutes.
- Wash the celery stalks. Cut the stalks into two to three-inch pieces and serve with the cream cheese.

FIRST COURSES

Keto Cauliflower and Spinach Super Soup

This soup is as nutritious as they come. It's creamy and it's Keto.

- Prep Time: 10 minutes
- Cooking time: 10 minutes
- Yields: Six servings

What you need:

- 1 medium cauliflower
- 2 garlic cloves
- 1 medium white or yellow onion
- 1 dried and crumbled bay leaf
- 200 grams of fresh spinach
- 150 grams of watercress
- 4 cups of vegetable broth
- 1 cup of coconut milk or dairy cream
- ¼ cup of ghee*
- 1 teaspoon salt
- Freshly ground black pepper to taste
- Fresh parsley for garnishing

** Ghee is clarified butter and you can purchase it at your local grocer, or it takes 15 minutes to make your own. You use 1 package (8.8 ounces) of unsalted butter with either a head of garlic or a medium onion of your choosing and your favorite herbs such as thyme, mint, rosemary, basil, sage, etc. Melt your butter slowly in a pan, then add the sliced garlic or diced onion and let it simmer. The milk solids will separate from the fat and any water will evaporate. After approximately 10 minutes the milk solids will stick to the pan and turn golden in color. Remove from heat and place a strainer over a heat resistant glass or jar. Cover the strainer with double cheesecloth* *and pour the ghee into the cheesecloth. Discard any milk solids and the garlic pieces remaining in the cheesecloth.*

What to do:

- Dice your garlic and onion finely. Place in a pan greased with ghee and sauté over medium heat until browned.
- Wash the spinach and watercress. Set aside.
- Cut your cauliflower into small florets and add to the browned onion. Add in the dried and crumbled bay leaf. Cook for approximately 5 minutes stirring often.
- Add the watercress and spinach and cook for another 2 to 3 minutes.
- Pour in your vegetable broth and bring the mixture to a boil. When the cauliflower is tender add the coconut milk. Add the salt and pepper. Remove from the heat and blend in a blender until creamy and smooth.
- Add fresh parsley for garnish.

Keto Cauliflower Cream Cheese Soup

This soup is the next best thing to creamy potato soup without the calories or the carbs. It's luscious, it's creamy, it's great tasting, and it's Keto.

- Prep Time: 10 minutes
- Cooking time: 20 minutes
- Yields: Five servings

What you need:

- 2 tablespoons butter
- ¼ small white or yellow onion
- 3 chopped garlic cloves
- 4 cups of grated cauliflower
- 1 tablespoon of fresh chopped dill
- 2 tablespoons of water
- 2 tablespoons of rice flour
- 1 ¾ cups of vegetable broth
- 2 cups of coconut milk
- 8 ounces of 1/3 less fat softened cream cheese (room temperature)
- ¾ teaspoon of salt
- Freshly ground black pepper to taste
- Fresh parsley for garnishing

What to do:

- Grate your cauliflower with a food processor or blender or a box grater. It should appear similar to rice. Set aside.

- In a sauce pan, sauté the chopped onion and garlic in 2 tablespoons of butter for 3 to 4 minutes until translucent and tender. Add in the grated cauliflower together with one tablespoon of fresh chopped dill, ¾ teaspoon of salt and a generous quantity of freshly ground black pepper. Blend well to cover all the cauliflower.
- Add in two tablespoons of water. Cover the pot and steam your cauliflower until tender. Stir several times.
- Now add in 2 cups of coconut milk, 1 ½ cups of vegetable broth and some more pepper. Raise the heat to medium high and allow the soup to bubble.
- Blend the remaining ¼ cup of vegetable broth with 2 tablespoons of rice flour and add slowly to the soup. Mix and simmer for 5 minutes until your soup has thickened somewhat.
- Now add in your cream cheese softened at room temperature. Once the cheese has been added, whisk the soup mixture thoroughly until all is amalgamated.
- Add salt and pepper to taste if so desired. Remove from the heat and allow to thicken, a little more before serving.

Keto Vegetarian Egg Drop Soup

This soup is incredibly easy and quick to make. In a pinch it's a great soup to serve on the spur of the moment for unexpected guests. Low carb, keto and satisfying.

- Prep Time: 10 minutes
- Cooking time: 10 minutes
- Yields: 5 servings

What you need:

- 4 ½ cups of vegetable broth
- 1/" cup of green onion, chopped
- 2 tablespoons of coconut aminos*
- ¼ teaspoon of ground ginger
- 2 eggs
- 1 egg yolk
- ½ teaspoon of salt
- ½ teaspoon of freshly ground black pepper
- 2 tablespoons of coconut flour

**Can be purchased at your local grocer or online*

What to do:

- In a large soup pan, heat the 4 cups of vegetable broth together with the chopped green onion, coconut aminos, ginger, salt and pepper bringing the mixture to a boil.
- In a smaller bowl combine the eggs and egg yolk together and whisk well. Now pour the eggs into the boiling broth and continue whisking to create strands of egg within the soup.

- In a smaller bowl mix together the remaining ¼ cup of vegetable broth and the two tablespoons of coconut flour. Whisk well and then whisk this mixture into your soup. Continue cooking for another 3 minutes until the soup thickens. Serve immediately while hot.

Keto Vegetarian Cream of Broccoli Soup

This is a totally awesome great tasting soup. And this low carb, keto recipe will allow you to thicken it without using flours or starches. The fresh cauliflower and broccoli are vitamin packed.

- Prep Time: 10 minutes
- Cooking time: 10 minutes
- Yields: 4 servings

What you need:

- 1 teaspoon of extra virgin olive oil
- 1 sliced medium white or yellow onion
- 1 teaspoon of salt
- Freshly ground black pepper to taste
- 4 cups of florets of cauliflower
- 3 cups of unsweetened almond milk
- 3 cups of finely chopped florets of broccoli
- 1 tablespoon of onion powder

What to do:

- In a large soup pan, add the olive oil, sliced onion, salt and pepper. Set the heat to medium high and sauté for at least five minutes. Add tablespoons of water as needed to avoid burning.
- Now add the cauliflower and the milk. Cover the pan and bring to a boil. Once your soup has been brought to a boil, reduce the heat and simmer covered for 10 minutes until all the florets are soft.
- Add half of the broccoli florets to the mixture.

- Now pour the mixture into your blender or food processor. Blend until smooth and creamy. Return to your soup pan.
- Blend in the remainder of the broccoli florets and the onion powder. Replace the lid and cook for 10 more minutes until thickened.
- Serve immediately while hot.

Keto Vegetarian Basil and Tomato Soup

A delicious low carb tomato soup that your whole family will enjoy.

- Prep Time: 2 to 3 minutes
- Cooking time: 10 minutes
- Yields: 6 servings

What you need:

- 1 can of whole plum tomatoes (28 ounces)
- 2 cups of water
- 1 tablespoon of butter
- 8 ounces of mascarpone cheese
- 2 tablespoons of granulated erythritol sweetener
- 1 ½ teaspoons of salt
- ½ teaspoon of onion powder
- ¼ teaspoon of garlic powder
- 1 teaspoon of apple cider vinegar
- ¼ teaspoon dried basil leaves
- ¼ cup of prepared basil pesto*

**You can prepare un quick and easy basil pesto with ¼ cup of olive oil, 2 tablespoons of pine nuts, 3 chopped garlic cloves, 1 cup of fresh basil leaves, ½ cup of fresh parsley, 1 tablespoon of fresh lemon juice, 2 teaspoons of yeast flakes, salt and freshly ground black pepper. Heat 1 teaspoon of oil add the pine nuts and garlic, sauté and set aside. Place the basil, parsley, yeast flakes, the remaining olive oil, the toasted pine nuts, garlic and lemon juice into a blender and blend. Season the pesto with salt and pepper to taste.*

What to do:

- Mix the canned tomatoes together with the water, salt, onion powder, and garlic powder in a saucepan.
- Bring the mixture to a boil on medium high heat and continue simmering for another 2 to 3 minutes.
- Remove from the stove and blend in a blender until creamy smooth. Return the mixture to the pan.
- Return the mixture to the stove over low heat. Now add the mascarpone and the butter to the soup mixture.
- Blend stirring over low heat for 2 to 3 minutes until creamy and until the cheese and butter are completely melted.
- Remove from the stove and stir in the apple cider vinegar, sweetener, dried basil and the pesto. Serve warm.

Keto Vegetarian Mushroom Risotto with Cauliflower Rice

This is an aromatic vegetarian substitute for risotto lovers looking for a low carb option. This recipe is quick and easy and very tasty. You can purchase frozen cauliflower rice or make your own by grating a medium head of cauliflower in your food processor. Whatever your choice, this vegetarian keto risotto will be a hit with whoever has the good fortune to be invited to your dinner table.

- Prep Time: 10 minutes
- Cooking time: 10 minutes
- Yields: 2 cups

What you need:

- 1 ½ cups mushrooms
- ½ cup of diced red onion
- 2 freshly crushed cloves of garlic
- 2 tablespoons of extra virgin olive oil
- 1 teaspoon salt
- 1 teaspoon freshly ground black pepper
- ½ teaspoon of ground sage
- 1 cup of coconut milk (13.5 ounces)
- 4 cups of cauliflower rice

What to do:

- Place a can of coconut milk in the refrigerator overnight.
- Prepare the onions and mushrooms, cutting them into small pieces.

- Place all of your ingredients into a skillet with the exception of the cauliflower rice and the coconut milk. Sauté on medium high heat until mushrooms and onions are soft.
- Take the can of coconut milk from the refrigerator, and once opened, remove only the top layer of hardened coconut fat. Do not use the coconut water.
- Place the hardened coconut fat and cauliflower rice into the skillet and mix together until well blended.
- Simmer over medium heat until the cauliflower rice is soft.
- Now add salt and pepper to taste and serve.

Keto Vegetarian Cheesy Cauliflower Risotto

This is a wonderful cheesy vegetarian substitute for risotto lovers looking for low carb options. Easy to fix, with quick prep and cooking times, this cauliflower risotto is an incredibly tasty offering especially for cheese lovers.

- Prep Time: 15 minutes
- Cooking time: 10 minutes
- Yields: 4 servings

What you need:

- 6 cups of cauliflower rice
- ¼ cup of butter
- 1 small finely chopped white onion
- 1 cup of vegetable broth
- 1 teaspoon of Dijon mustard
- 1 cup of shredded cheddar cheese
- 1 cup of grated Parmesan cheese
- 4 tablespoons of chopped fresh chives
- Salt to taste

What to do:

- Purchase frozen cauliflower rice or make your own by grating a large head of cauliflower in your food processor or blender until rice like in size and consistency.
- Grease a large skillet with the butter. Once the pan is hot, sauté the chopped onion over medium heat until brown.
- Now add the cauliflower rice and blend well. Cook for several minutes and then add the vegetable broth. Cook for at least

five minutes until the cauliflower is tender. While cooking, grate the cheddar and Parmesan cheese.

- Add in the mustard, stirring, and remove form the stove.
- Add the grated cheeses and blend well. Keep a little Parmesan aside to garnish. Do the same with the fresh chives, adding and blending, with some chives set aside for the garnish. Salt to taste.
- Transfer the "Risotto" Into serving dishes and garnish with Parmesan and chives.

Keto Vegetarian Zucchini Noodles with Avocado Sauce

If you love spaghetti but don't want the carbs, zoodles or zucchini noodles are your answer. And these zucchini noodles with a luscious avocado sauce are ready in ten minutes flat. It can't get any easier for such a great dish.

- Prep Time: 10 minutes
- Yields: 2 servings

What you need:

- 1 zucchini
- 1 ¼ cup of fresh basil
- 1/3 cup of water
- 4 tablespoons of pine nuts
- 2 tablespoons of lemon juice
- 1 avocado
- 12 cherry tomatoes, sliced

What to do:

- Make your zucchini noodles using a peeler or a "spiralizer". *
- Mix in a blender, the basil, water, pine nuts, lemon juice and the avocado until very smooth.
- Now mix the zucchini noodles, avocado sauce and the sliced cherry tomatoes together in a mixing bowl.
- Serve fresh.

**A "spiralizer" is a spiral vegetable slicer, which can be purchased in cooking supplies stores or on line.*

Keto Vegetarian Spinach and Zucchini Lasagna

You love pasta. You love lasagna and you feel guilty. Really guilty. Now you can enjoy guilt-free zucchini lasagna, which is low carb, vegetarian and keto-friendly. Best of all, it tastes great!

- Prep Time: 20 minutes
- Cooking Time: 50 minutes
- Yields: 9 servings

What you need:

- 1 tablespoon extra-virgin olive oil
- ½ finely chopped white or yellow onion
- 4 crushed garlic cloves
- 2 tablespoons of tomato paste
- 1 ¾ lbs. of fresh tomatoes which have been peeled, seeded and diced
- 1 tablespoon fresh chopped basil
- 3 cups of spinach
- 15 ounces of partially skimmed ricotta
- 1 egg
- ½ cup of grated Parmesan cheese
- 4 medium sized zucchinis
- 16 ounces of partly skimmed shredded mozzarella cheese
- ½ teaspoon of parsley
- Salt to taste
- Ground black pepper to taste

What to do:

- Heat the olive oil in a saucepan over medium high heat.

- Place the onions in the pan and cook for 5 minutes until translucent and soft.
- Mix in the garlic and sauté without burning.
- Add in the tomato paste and blend well. Now add in the tomatoes.
- Season with salt and black pepper.
- Cover the pan and simmer for about 30 minutes.
- Remove from the stove and mix in the fresh basil and spinach, stirring well.
- Preheat your oven to 375° Fahrenheit.
- Slice the zucchini into 1/8 of an inch slice. Arrange the slices in a layer on a baking sheet and paint with olive oil. Broil for 8 minutes. Remove from your oven, cool, and eliminate any excess moisture with paper towels.
- In a bowl, combine the ricotta and Parmesan cheeses with an egg stirring well.
- In a casserole dish sized 9" X 15" paint the bottom with the tomato and spinach sauce. Then cover with 5 to 6 zucchini slices. Place a layer of ricotta cheese mixture and top with shredded mozzarella. Repeat all these layers until you have used up all of your ingredients. Complete by topping with sauce and mozzarella.
- Cover the baking dish with aluminum foil and bake for 30 minutes. Then uncover and bake for another 15 minutes.
- Allow the lasagna to cool for about ten minutes and garnish with fresh parsley. Serve and enjoy.

Keto Vegetarian Snap Pea Salad

This Keto Snap Pea Salad is a refreshing springtime dish, appetizing and tasty for either lunch or dinner.

- Prep Time: 15 minutes
- Cooking time: 12 minutes
- Yields: 4 servings

What you need:

- 6 ounces of cauliflower rice
- ¼ cup of lemon juice
- ¼ cup of olive oil
- 1 crushed garlic clove
- ½ teaspoon of Dijon mustard
- 1 teaspoon of granulated sweetener (Combo of stevia and erythritol)
- ¼ teaspoon of pepper
- ½ teaspoon salt
- ½ cup of sugar snap peas*
- ¼ cup of chives
- ½ cup of sliced almonds
- ¼ cup of minced red onions

The peas should have the ends removed, and each of the pods should be cut into three equal pieces.

What to do:

- Pour 2 inches of water into a pot with a steamer inside. Allow the water to simmer.

- Place the cauliflower rice in the steaming basket, sprinkle with a pinch of salt, cover and place over the simmering water in the bottom of the steamer pot. Proceed steaming until tender for approximately 12 minutes.
- Once the cauliflower is tender, remove the top of the steamer from the water, which is simmering and place in a bowl so any excess water can drain. Set aside and cool. Once cooled, cover and place both steamer and bowl into the refrigerator. Chill for a half an hour.
- While cooling the cauliflower, proceed to prepare the dressing. Pour the olive oil in a bowl and gradually add in the lemon juice, whisking. Then whisk in the Dijon mustard, garlic, pepper, salt and the sweetener.
- In a larger bowl, mix the chilled cauliflower rice, peas, almonds, chives, and the red onions. Pour on the dressing and toss gently. The salad should be refrigerated for several hours before serving.

Keto Vegetarian Greek Salad

This Keto Greek Salad is as good tasting as you'll find in any restaurant. Easy and quick to toss together, this salad will delight at either lunch or dinner.

- Prep Time: 10 minutes
- Cooking time: 0 minutes
- Yields: 6 servings

What you need:

- 2 peeled and chopped cucumbers
- 1 pint of grape tomatoes which have been halved
- 4 ounces of cubed feta cheese
- 2 tablespoons of fresh dill
- 2 tablespoons of extra virgin olive oil

What to do:

- Combine and mix the cucumbers, tomatoes, feta cheese and dill in a bowl, tossing gently. Drizzle the ingredients with olive oil and continue tossing to mix.
- Serve.

Keto Vegetarian Fried Goat Cheese with Charred veggies Salad

This Keto Greek Salad is as good tasting as you'll find in any restaurant. Easy and quick to toss together, this salad will delight at either lunch or dinner.

- Prep Time: 10 minutes
- Cooking time: 5 to 10 minutes
- Yields: 2 servings

What you need:

- 2 tablespoons of poppy seeds
- 2 tablespoons of sesame seeds
- 1 teaspoon of onion flakes
- 1 teaspoon of garlic flakes
- 4 ounces of goat cheeses cut into four ½ inch thick medallions
- 1 medium sized red pepper, seeded and cut into 8 pieces
- ½ cup of mushrooms
- 4 cups of arugula divided between 2 salad plates
- 1 tablespoon of avocado oil

What to do:

- Combine and mix the poppy seeds, sesame seeds, onion flakes, and garlic flakes in a bowl.

- Cover the four pieces of goat cheese with the mix on both sides. Refrigerate until it is time to fry the cheese.
- Prepare a frying pan, spraying it with nonstick cooking spray and heat on medium to high. Now char the peppers and mushrooms on each side until they darken, and the pepper should soften. Now add the mushrooms and pepper to the plates with the arugula.
- Now place the chilled goat cheese into the frying pan and fry on each side. As the cheese melts quickly, it must be handled and flipped with care.
- Now add to the cheese to the salad plates and sprinkle with the avocado oil. Serve while the cheese is warm.

MAIN COURSES

Cauliflower Parmesan Steak

For KETO vegetarians, this entrée offers a delightful option made of fresh vegetable with contrasting textures for followers of plant-based diets. Low carb, with the right mix of seasoning you'll have a savory dinner to enjoy.

- Prep Time:
- Cooking time:
- Yields: 4 servings

What you need:

- 1 head of cauliflower
- 4 tablespoons of butter
- 2 tablespoons of seasoning*
- ¼ cup of Parmesan cheese, grated
- Salt and pepper as needed

** In a bowl mix together ½ teaspoon pepper, 1 teaspoon salt, ½ teaspoon garlic powder and ½ teaspoon paprika for your seasoning mix.*

What to do:

- Preheat your oven to 400° Fahrenheit.
- Remove any leaves from your cauliflower.
- Slice your cauliflower lengthwise into at least one-inch thick steaks. Slice through the core.
- Melt the butter in a microwave and mix with your seasonings to create a paste.

- Brush your cauliflower steaks with the paste. Add salt and pepper to your taste.
- Heat a nonstick frying pan over medium heat and brown lightly the cauliflower steaks on both sides.
- Now place the browned cauliflower steaks on a lined baking sheet and bake for 20 minutes.
- Remove from the oven, and sprinkle with Parmesan. Serve immediately.

Keto Fried Goat Cheese

If you've never tried fried goat cheese, this is your chance. This recipe provides cheese medallions that are crunchy and crispy on the outside with a soft creamy heart. Every bite offers distinctive tasteful flavor.

- Prep Time: 10 minutes
- Cooking time: 3 minutes
- Yields: 4 servings

What you need:

- 1 ounce of ground smoked tofu
- 8 ounces of goat cheese, (Cheese log) chilled
- 2 eggs
- ½ teaspoon of dried parsley flakes
- ¼ teaspoon of salt
- ½ cup of coconut flour
- 1 ½ cups of coconut oil for frying

What to do:

- Place the coconut oil in a saucepan and set the heat to medium high. Put a thermometer in the oil to check the temperature periodically.
- Put the coconut flour in a small bowl. In a second bowl whisk the eggs and put the ground, smoked tofu into a third bowl.
- Slice your log of goat cheese into 8 separate medallions. Lay them on a plate and set aside.

- Individually coat each slice of goat cheese in the coconut flour, followed by the whisked eggs, and then in the smoked tofu. Return to the plate.
- When your coconut oil reaches 345° place two of your medallions into the oil and fry for about half a minute. Gently turn the cheese over and fry the other side for another half minute. Remove and place on a paper towel to remove excess oil. When you have fried all the cheese, serve.

Roasted Caprese Tomatoes with Basil Dressing

If you enjoy a good Italian caprese salad, you'll delight in these roasted caprese tomatoes. The wonderful taste of fresh tomatoes is enhanced during the roasting and literally permeates the cheese creating an explosion of flavor with every bite.

- Prep Time: 5 minutes
- Cooking time: 30 minutes
- Yields: 2 to 4 servings

What you need:

- 4 large tomatoes, ripe
- 1 tablespoon of extra virgin olive oil
- 2 tablespoons of balsamic vinegar
- 4 slices of mozzarella, sliced thinly
- 4 fresh basil leaves

For the basil dressing:

- A fistful of fresh basil
- 1 clove of garlic
- The juice of ½ lemon
- 2 tablespoons of extra virgin olive oil
- Salt as needed

What to do:

- Preheat your oven to 350° Fahrenheit/180° Celsius.

- Slice your tomatoes in halves and place them on a nonstick baking sheet with the cut side facing up.
- Sprinkle some olive oil, balsamic vinegar, salt and pepper.
- Now roast for about 25 minutes. The skins should be blistered. Place a slice of mozzarella cheese on top of each tomato and continue roasting for 5 more minutes.
- Remove from the oven. On each bottom half, place a fresh basil leaf. Now rejoin the two tomato halves.
- Blend the dressing ingredients in your blender or food processor until the fresh basil is very finely chopped.
- Serve your roasted tomatoes warm sprinkled with dressing.

Vegetarian Cauliflower crust Pizza with Mushrooms and Olives

If you're a vegetarian keto follower who likes pizza, this cauliflower crust alternative may very well satisfy your desire for some. It can be cooked using a pizza stone or in your oven. And the cauliflower crust gives you an extra helping of vegetables.

- Prep Time: 25 minutes
- Cooking time: 20 minutes
- Yields: 2 servings

What you need for your crust:

- 1 cup of very finely chopped cauliflower
- ½ cup of low-fat mozzarella cheese, finely grated
- 5 tablespoons of almond meal
- 3 tablespoons of Parmesan cheese, finely grated
- 1 teaspoon of dried oregano flakes
- ½ teaspoon of garlic powder
- A pinch of salt
- 1 beaten egg

For your pizza topping:

- ¼ cup of tomato sauce
- 3 tablespoons of mozzarella cheese, finely grated
- 2 tablespoons of extra virgin olive oil
- 4 ounces of mushrooms that have been sliced and sautéed
- ¼ cup of olives, halved

What to do:

- Preheat your oven to 450° Fahrenheit/230° Celsius. If you have a pizza stone place it inside. If you are not using a pizza stone, heat the oven a little higher.
- Now using a food processor, blender or box grater, chop the cauliflower into bits that resemble rice.
- Place the cauliflower in a microwave safe bowl and cook the cauliflower until it's completely softened (about 8 minutes). Do not add any water or liquid.
- While you wait for the cauliflower to cook, slice your mushrooms and sauté them in a skillet with the olive oil. They should be well cooked and soft.
- Slice all of your olives lengthwise in half. Pulse your mozzarella cheese in your food processor or blender to grate it as finely as possible.
- In a bowl, mix the cooked cauliflower with the almond meal, Parmesan cheese, ½ cup of the finely grated mozzarella, oregano flakes, garlic powder and the pinch of salt. Whisk the egg and add it to the other ingredients making sure to blend well.
- Now spray a cookie sheet with nonstick cooking spray.
- Roll the crust dough into a ball and place it on your cookie sheet. Now work the crust with your fingers to spread it as thin as possible. Put the cookie sheet on the pizza stone or directly in the oven and cook for about 15 minutes, or until the crust is firm and golden.
- When your crust is ready, spread on the tomato sauce, sprinkle on the cheese and distribute your sautéed mushrooms and olives evenly.

- Return the pizza to the oven to melt the cheese and warm your toppings. You can use the broiler and cook for 3 to 5 minutes. Serve hot.

Keto Roasted Baby Eggplant with Ricotta

In Italy, eggplant is a staple throughout the country. And if there's one thing the Italians know well, it's food. This delightful vegetable coupled with creamy ricotta cheese will delight your palate for both taste and texture.

- Prep Time: 5 minutes
- Cooking time: 45 minutes
- Yields: 16 halves

What you need:

- 8 baby eggplants
- 1 teaspoon of wild fennel
- 2 tablespoons of extra virgin olive oil
- 1 teaspoon of salt
- 1 teaspoon of black pepper
- 1/3 cup of fresh ricotta cheese
- 2 more tablespoons of extra virgin olive oil
- Black pepper, freshly ground
- Salt

What to do:

- Preheat your oven to 350° Fahrenheit/180° Celsius.
- Wash the eggplants and slice them into halves. Place them on a cookie sheet with the cut side facing upward. Sprinkle some olive oil on the cut halves followed by the fennel, salt and pepper.
- Place in your oven and bake for 45 minutes. The eggplant should be soft and slightly browned. Remove the eggplant

from the oven and allow to cool. Add on a generous teaspoon of ricotta on each half. Grind some black pepper corns and a pinch of salt. Now drizzle on a bit of olive oil. Enjoy the delicious filling, while avoiding eating the skin, which remains somewhat tough.

Keto Vegetarian Mexican Cauliflower Patties

These cauliflower patties are so very tasty, that you'll never have leftovers. A great entrée for lunch or dinner or maybe even a snack, they are vegetarian and gluten free.

- Prep Time: 15 minutes
- Cooking time: 10 minutes
- Yields: 8 patties

What you need:

- 1 head of cauliflower, chopped into large florets
- 3 minced scallions
- 2 beaten eggs
- ¼ cup of cilantro, chopped
- ¼ cup of almond flour
- 1 tablespoon of Mexican spices*
- ¼ teaspoon of salt
- 1 cup of sharp cheddar cheese, shredded
- 2 tablespoons of coconut oil
- lime wedges

**You can make your own batch of Mexican seasoning by combining a tablespoon of ground cumin, dried coriander flakes, and mild paprika, with a teaspoon of dried oregano flakes, ½ teaspoon of chili powder and of garlic powder.*

What to do:

- Boil several inches of water in a saucepan with a steamer basket inside. Preheat your oven to 300° Fahrenheit. Spray a baking sheet with nonstick cooking spray.
- Place the cauliflower in the steamer basket, cover and steam for 8 minutes or until the cauliflower is tender. Remove the basket and allow the cauliflower to cool for at least 10 minutes.
- While waiting, combine the scallions, eggs, cilantro, almond flower, salt and spices together in a bowl.
- Puree the cauliflower in your blender or food processor until it is paste-like. It should not be smooth but seem more like rice bits. Add this cauliflower to the spice mix and blend really well. Finally add in the cheddar combine together well.
- Heat 1 tablespoon of oil in a skillet over medium-heat. Separate the mixture into 8 portions and prepare 8 patty mounds. Place four cauliflower mounds in the skillet and cover to cook, being careful not to scorch or burn the patties. Only flip the patties in order to brown both sides when they will not break apart. As you cook the patties, keep them warm in your oven until serving. Repeat the procedure for the second group of four patties.
- Serve warm with lime wedges.

Keto Indian Egg Curry

If you enjoy Indian food or any curry dish, you'll enjoy this keto version of Indian egg curry. It's savory and spicy and mouthwatering.

- Prep Time: 10 minutes
- Cooking time: 10 minutes
- Yields: 2 servings

What you need:

- 4 eggs boiled
- 50 grams of onion
- 100 grams of tomato
- 10 grams of ginger
- 5 grams of garlic
- 1 green chilly
- 1 tablespoon of ghee
- Coriander for garnishing
- Salt
- ¼ teaspoon of turmeric
- ½ teaspoon of red chili powder
- ½ teaspoon of coriander powder
- ¼ teaspoon of Garam Masala

What to do:

- Allow the eggs to reach room temperature and then place in a pan of boiling water for about 6 minutes.
- Peel the eggs and set aside.

- Mix a paste by combining the onion, garlic, ginger and chilly together.
- Puree the tomato.
- Heat the ghee in a pan and fry the onion, ginger, garlic and chili paste until browned.
- Add the turmeric, coriander powder, chilli powder and garam masala to the mixture.
- Cook for two minutes and pour in the tomato puree, water and salt. Cover and simmer for 10 minutes.
- Now add in the eggs and cook for another 2 to 3 minutes.
- Garnish with fresh coriander and serve.

Keto Cheesy Cauliflower alla Vodka casserole

Vodka sauce for pasta is quite well known in American-Italian restaurants. When you follow a keto diet, that pasta option goes out the window. So if you've missed your pasta with vodka sauce, now you can try this delicate cauliflower casserole alla vodka without feeling too guilty.

- Prep Time: 10 minutes
- Cooking time: 40 minutes
- Yields: 8 servings

What you need:

- 8 cups of cauliflower florets
- 2 cups of vodka sauce*
- 2 tablespoons of heavy whipping cream
- 2 tablespoons of butter, melted
- 1/3 cup of Parmesan cheese, grated
- ½ teaspoon salt
- ¼ teaspoon black pepper
- 6 slices of Provolone cheese
- ¼ cup of chopped fresh basil

**The vodka sauce can be purchased, or home made. To make a homemade sauce pour a 35-ounce can of Italian plum tomatoes with their liquid into your food processor or blender and pulse until finely chopped, not pureed. Heat a ¼ cup of extra virgin olive oil in a skillet and sauté 10 garlic cloves for 3 minutes. Now add the tomatoes into the skillet, bringing to a boil seasoning with salt and hot crushed red pepper. Boil for 2 minutes. Pour in ¼ cup of vodka and lower the heat to simmer for several minutes. Remove* *the garlic cloves and add in ½ cup of heavy cream. Add in another 2 tablespoons of olive oil to complete the sauce.*

What to do:

- Preheat your oven to 375° Fahrenheit.
- Mix together the cauliflower, vodka sauce, whipping cream, Parmesan cheese, butter, salt, and pepper in a large bowl making sure to mix well and coat the cauliflower.
- Pour the mixture into a 9" x 13" baking dish and top with the slices of Provolone cheese.
- Bake for 40 minutes. The casserole should bubble, and the cheese should be melted completely.
- Remove from the oven and let it cool for about 10 minutes.
- Garnish with the chopped fresh basil and serve.

Keto Vegetarian Sesame Tofu and Eggplant

This delightful sesame and tofu entrée is an appetizing light dish that is great for lunch or dinner. This recipe stars eggplant in a spicy marinade sauce coupled with tofu that's sesame seed crusted and seared. Yummy.

- Prep Time: 20 minutes
- Cooking time: 20 to 30 minutes
- Yields: 4 servings

What you need:

- 1 lb. block of tofu
- 1 cup of chopped fresh cilantro
- 3 tablespoons of rice vinegar
- 4 tablespoons of toasted sesame oil
- 2 finely minced garlic cloves
- 1 teaspoon of crushed red pepper flakes
- 2 teaspoons of a sweetener of choice
- 1 eggplant about 450 grams
- 1 tablespoon of extra virgin olive oil
- Salt and pepper as needed
- ¼ cup of sesame seeds
- ¼ cup of soy sauce

What to do:

- Preheat your oven to 200° Fahrenheit. Wrap the tofu block in paper towels and place a heavy plate on top to press any excess water from the tofu.
- In a large mixing bowl, combine ¼ cup of cilantro, the rice vinegar, minced garlic, 2 tablespoons of sesame oil, crushed

red pepper flakes and the sweetener and whisk everything together.

- Peel the eggplant and julienne it by hand or with a mandolin. Place the eggplant julienne noodles into the marinade mixture.
- Place a frying pan over medium to low heat and add in a tablespoon of olive oil. Cook the eggplant until it is soft.
- Now turn off the oven. Mix the remaining cilantro into the eggplant noodles, then transfer the noodles to an oven safe dish. Cover with aluminum foil and place in the oven in order to keep warm. Clean the frying pan and return it to the stove to continue cooking.
- Unwrap your tofu block and slice into 8 pieces. Place the sesame seeds on a platter and press both sides of the tofu slices into the seeds.
- Add in 2 tablespoons of the sesame oil to the frying pan. Fry the tofu on both sides for 5 minutes on each side. They should become crispy. Add a ¼ cup of soy sauce into the frying pan and coat the tofu slices. Continue cooking until the tofu is golden brown and the soy sauce has caramelized.
- Remove the noodles from the oven and place the tofu on top of the eggplant noodles and serve.

Keto Low Carb Fried Mac and Cheese

If you loved traditional Mac and Cheese before following Keto, you'll be delighted by this keto friendly version that doesn't interfere with your new keto lifestyle. This dish is tasty, tempting, and as satisfying as comfort food can be.

- Prep Time: 15 minutes
- Cooking time: 15 minutes
- Yields: 8 to 10 patties

What you need:

- 1 medium cauliflower, to make cauliflower rice
- 1 ½ cups of cheddar cheese, shredded
- 3 eggs
- 2 teaspoons of paprika
- 1 teaspoon of turmeric
- ¾ teaspoon of dried rosemary

What to do:

- Cut the cauliflower and form florets. Now put these florets in a food processor or blender and blend until the cauliflower appears like rice bits.
- Place the riced cauliflower in a microwave safe dish and microwave the cauliflower rice for 7 minutes. When the microwaving is completed place the cauliflower in paper towels and press to remove any excess moisture. After pressing out the excess moisture return the cauliflower to a bowl.

- Add the eggs one at a time to the riced cauliflower, then proceed to add the cheese, followed by the turmeric, rosemary and the paprika. Blend the mixture very well to get a good balance of the ingredients.
- In a pan, heat the olive oil and the coconut oil over a high heat until very, very hot. Turn portions of the cauliflower mixture into balls. Then pat the balls into patties.
- Place the patties in the oil and reduce the heat to medium to cook. They should become crispy brown on one side before flipping. Repeat, cooking the other side. Now serve with a side dish of your choosing. Enjoy!

SIDE DISHES

Easy Keto Cheese Zucchini Gratin

Zucchini is a great vegetable side dish to complete your KETO meal. For a delicious twist, try this easy cheese zucchini dish that even Keto haters will absolutely love.

- Prep Time: 10 minutes
- Cooking time: 50 minutes
- Yields: 9 servings

What you need:

- 4 cups of raw zucchini sliced
- 1 small yellow or white medium onion that should be sliced thinly
- 1 ½ cups of pepper jack cheese, shredded
- 2 tablespoons of butter
- ½ teaspoon of garlic powder
- ¼ teaspoon of xanthan gum
- Salt to taste
- Ground black pepper to taste
- ½ cup of heavy whipping cream

What to do:

- Preheat your oven to 375° Fahrenheit. Grease a 9 x 9-inch baking pan.
- Place a third of the zucchini and onion slices into the pan overlapping them. Season with salt and pepper to taste and sprinkle ½ cup of the pepper jack cheese on top.

- Repeat this until you have formed three layers and all of the zucchini, cheese and onion have been employed.
- In a microwave dish, mix the garlic powder, heavy cream, xanthan gum and butter together.
- Heat in the microwave for about a minute until the butter is melted and then whisk the mixture until it's smooth.
- Pour the butter mixture over the zucchini and onion layers.
- Bake in your over for 45 to 50 minutes. The top should be golden brown.
- Serve while warm.

Keto Vegetarian Stuffed Zucchini with Goat Cheese and Tomato Sauce

This is a really easy zucchini side dish where the great taste seems like you put much more work into it. Quick to make with only three ingredients it will make a wonderful complement to your dinner meal.

- Prep Time: 10 minutes
- Cooking time: 12 minutes
- Yields: 4 servings

What you need:

- 4 medium zucchinis
- 15 ounces of goat cheese
- 1 to 2 cups of tomato or marinara sauce
- Fresh parsley, chopped for garnish

What to do:

- Preheat your oven to 400° Fahrenheit.
- Cut your zucchini lengthwise in half and clean out the seeds, leaving a hollow zucchini shell. Season your zucchini shell with salt and pepper and place on a baking sheet or in an appropriately sized baking dish.
- Take half of the goat cheese and place some in each zucchini, then place some tomato or marinara sauce on top. Now place the remaining goat cheese on top.

- You can bake or grill your zucchini for approximately 10 to 12 minutes until the goat cheese melts and the tomato sauce bubbles.
- Serve hot.

Keto Vegetarian Eggplant Gratin with Feta

Luscious cream covering tasty eggplant steeped in herbs and salty feta cheese. This side dish may very well steal the show. It's a party for your taste buds.

- Prep Time: 10 minutes
- Cooking time: 12 minutes
- Yields: 4 servings

What you need:

- 1 eggplant about 30 ounces in weight
- 2 white or yellow onions
- 2 tablespoons of extra virgin olive oil
- 5.3 ounces of feta cheese
- 1 tablespoon of mint, dried or freshly chopped
- 1/3 cup of finely chopped fresh parsley
- 4 ounces of grated Parmesan cheese
- ¾ cup of heavy whipping cream
- Salt to taste
- Freshly ground black pepper

What to do:

- Preheat your oven to 400° Fahrenheit (200° Celsius)
- Cut the eggplant into half inch-thick slices.
- Paint the slices on both sides with olive oil and salt and place on a lined baking sheet.
- Bake in your oven until golden.

- While baking, slice the onion into thin slices with your food processor or a mandoline.
- Sauté the onion in a skillet with olive oil over medium heat until translucent and soft. Season with salt and black pepper to taste.
- Put a layer of baked eggplant into a baking pan, then a layer of onions followed by mint, parsley and two thirds of the feta cheese. Add on a final layer of baked eggplant and the onion. Finish with the remaining feta cheese and grated Parmesan cheese as a topping.
- Pour the cream over the ingredients. Bake in the oven at 450 ° Fahrenheit for 30 minutes until the cream bubbles and the gratin is golden.

Keto Garlic and Chive Cauliflower Mash

A delicious dairy free cauliflower puree that is low carb and very keto friendly.

- Prep Time: 10 minutes
- Cooking time: 12 minutes
- Yields: 4 servings

What you need:

- 4 cups of cauliflower cut into florets
- 1/3 cup of mayonnaise
- 1 garlic clove
- 1 tablespoon of water
- ½ teaspoon of salt
- 1/8 teaspoon of black pepper freshly ground
- ¼ teaspoon of lemon juice
- ½ teaspoon of lemon zest
- 1 tablespoon of chopped fresh chives

What to do:

- Mix the florets of cauliflower, garlic, mayonnaise, water, salt and pepper in a microwave safe bowl, stirring to make sure the florets are coated. Now microwave the mixture on high for about 15 minutes making sure that the cauliflower is completely softened.
- Place the mixture in your blender or food processor and puree until creamy smooth.

- Add in the lemon juice, lemon zest and fresh chives and pulse until well blended.
- Serve warm.

Keto Creamy Cilantro Lime Coleslaw

This keto coleslaw is low carb and perfect for summer meals or to complete a wonderful grilled vegetarian lunch or supper. Wonderfully flavorful, crunchy and creamy!

- Prep Time: 10 minutes
- Cooking time: 0 minutes
- Yields: 5 servings

What you need:

- 14 ounces of bagged pre-shredded coleslaw mix
- 1 ½ ripe avocados
- ¼ cup of cilantro leaves
- Juice of 2 limes
- 1 clove of garlic
- ¼ cup of water
- ½ teaspoon of salt
- Fresh cilantro for your garnish

What to do:

- Place the ¼ cup of cilantro leaves and the garlic in your blender or food processor until completely chopped.
- Add in the lime juice together with the avocados and water and pulse until creamy and smooth.
- Place your mixture in a good-sized bowl and mix it together with your pre-shredded coleslaw. Toss gently so that all of the slaw is covered in the cream.

- Refrigerate for several hours before eating.

Keto Eggplant fries

If you're craving French fries, this low carb eggplant recipe may satisfy those cravings. You can dip them, and they crunch!

- Prep Time: 10 minutes
- Cooking time: 10 minutes
- Yields: 4 to 6 servings

What you need:

- 2 eggplants, large
- 2 beaten eggs
- ½ cup of coconut flour
- ½ teaspoon of garlic powder
- ½ teaspoon of parsley flakes
- ½ cup of Parmesan cheese, grated
- 1/8 teaspoon of salt
- 1/8 teaspoon of ground black pepper
- ½ cup of extra virgin olive oil

What to do:

- Peel your 2 eggplants and cut them into strips that measure approximately ¾" wide and 4 inches in length to look like French fries.
- Beat the 2 eggs in a bowl.
- In a separate bowl, mix together the Parmesan cheese, garlic powder, coconut flour, parsley flakes, salt, and pepper.
- Begin heating the olive oil in a pan for sautéing.

- Coat the eggplant well with the egg mixture and then coat with the Parmesan and herb mixture.
- Once you have coated your eggplant strips, cook them in small groups in the hot oil, making sure to brown them on all sides. Remove them onto paper towels to absorb excess oil.

Serve with a low carb sauce of your choosing.

Keto Moroccan Roasted Green Beans

After tasting this savory and spicy side dish, you'll never think of green beans in the same manner again. Absolutely delish!

- Prep Time: 5 minutes not including the trimming of the green beans
- Cooking time: 30 minutes
- Yields: 6 servings

What you need:

- 6 cups of raw trimmed green beans
- 1 teaspoon of salt
- ½ teaspoon of black pepper
- 2 tablespoons of extra virgin olive oil
- 1 tablespoon of Ras el Hanout seasoning*

**This seasoning mix can be purchased, or home made. To make your own combine the following ground spices: 1 teaspoon of cumin, 1 teaspoon of ginger, ½ teaspoon of cinnamon, ½ coriander seeds, ½ teaspoon of allspice, ½ teaspoon of cayenne, ¼ teaspoon of cloves, ¾ teaspoon of black pepper, and 1 teaspoon of salt. Transfer to an airtight jar. These spices can be kept up to a month.*

What to do:

- Preheat your oven to 400° Fahrenheit (200° Celsius).
- Mix the olive oil and the seasonings together. Now toss the green beans with the oil mixture well.

- Spread the green beans onto a large baking sheet or in a large roasting pan.
- Roast the green beans for 20 minutes.
- Remove the green beans from the oven and stir well.
- Return the beans to the oven and roast them for 10 more minutes.
- Remove and serve. They can be served warm or chilled.

Keto Low carb Zucchini and Sweet potato Latkes

After tasting this savory and spicy side dish, you'll never think of green beans in the same manner again. Absolutely delish!

- Prep Time: 10 minutes
- Cooking time: 10 minutes
- Yields: 4 servings

What you need:

- 1 cup of zucchini, shredded
- 1 cup of sweet potato, shredded
- 1 whisked egg
- ½ teaspoon of garlic powder
- ¼ teaspoon of cumin, ground
- ½ teaspoon of dried parsley flakes
- 1 tablespoon of coconut flour
- 1 tablespoon of extra virgin olive oil
- 1 tablespoon of clarified butter or ghee
- Salt and pepper to taste

What to do:

- Mix together the zucchini, egg and sweet potato in a bowl.
- In a second bowl, combine the coconut flour and the various spices. Now add these dry ingredients to the sweet potato and zucchini mixture. Blend very well.
- Heat your olive oil and ghee in a medium sized pan that is nonstick. Separate your zucchini mixture into 4 separate

portions. Drop one of the 4 portions into the pan and press flat with a fork or metal spatula. Cook over medium heat until crisp and golden. Flip to cook on both sides. When cooked, place on a plate with paper towels to remove excess oil. Serve hot.

Keto Spinach and Artichoke Stuffed Mushrooms

With super healthy spinach and great tasting artichokes, these stuffed mushroom caps are a stellar side dish to serve with just about any vegetarian main course. Thoroughly delightful.

- Prep Time: 10 minutes
- Cooking time: 20 minutes
- Yields: 8 servings/each serving is half of a mushroom cap

What you need:

- 2 tablespoons of olive oil, preferably extra virgin
- 4 medium sized mushrooms with their stems and gills removed
- 1 10-ounce package of frozen spinach, cooked and drained
- 1 14 ounce can of artichoke hearts which should be drained and chopped
- 4 ounces of room temperature cream cheese
- ½ cup of Parmesan cheese grated
- 2 tablespoons of sour cream
- 2 chopped garlic cloves
- 3 ounces of shredded mozzarella cheese
- Salt and pepper as needed

What to do:

- Brush your mushroom caps with olive oil and place on a baking sheet. Broil on high for approximately 5 minutes on either side.

- Preheat your oven to 375° Fahrenheit.
- Remove any excess liquid from your cooked spinach by squeezing in paper towels.
- In a bowl, combine the artichoke pieces, spinach, garlic, cream cheese, Parmesan cheese, sour cream, salt, and pepper and blend well.
- Stuff your mushroom caps evenly with this mixture. Sprinkle some shredded mozzarella cheese on each caplet.
- Bake your mushroom caps in the preheated oven for approximately 15 minutes. *
- Serve.

**If you need to brown your mozzarella cheese topping, use the broiler for the final minute or two of your cooking time.*

Keto Three Cheese Quiche Stuffed Peppers

Keto Vegetarians will love these delectable peppers with cheese. This is probably the easiest quiche recipe available. Fluffy and delicious with good, rich cheese in a colorful pepper!

- Prep Time: 10 minutes
- Cooking time: 48 minutes
- Yields: 4 servings/each serving is half of a pepper

What you need:

- 2 Bell Peppers
- 4 large eggs
- 1 teaspoon of garlic powder
- ½ cup of Parmesan cheese, grated
- 2 tablespoons of Parmesan cheese
- ½ cup of Mozzarella cheese, shredded
- ½ cup of ricotta cheese
- ¼ teaspoon of dried parsley flakes
- ¼ cup of spinach

What to do:

- Preheat your oven to 375° Fahrenheit.
- Prepare your bell peppers by halving them and removing the seeds.
- Blend the ½ cups of the three cheeses in your blender or food processor together with the garlic powder, eggs and parsley.

- Now pour the mixture into the four pepper halves just below the rim. Place a few spinach leaves on top and stir into the egg mixture in the pepper.
- Cover the four pepper halves with aluminum foil and bake for about 45 minutes. The egg should set.
- Sprinkle the extra 2 tablespoons of Parmesan cheese on top and broil until the tops are golden brown.

DESSERTS

Keto Vegetarian Coconut Macaroons

Yummy Keto cookies that are sugar free and low carb. What more can you ask for?

- Prep Time: 20 minutes
- Cooking time: 25 minutes
- Yields: Twelve servings

What you need:

- 2 ½ cups of shredded unsweetened coconut
- ½ cup of almond flour
- ½ cup of erythritol or monk fruit sweetener
- 1 teaspoon of almond extract
- ½ cup of aquafaba (which is the liquid found in canned chickpeas)
- A pinch of salt
- ½ cup of sugar-free, dairy-free dark chocolate chips (o 90% dark chocolate that are dairy-free)

What to do:

- Preheat your oven to 350° Fahrenheit and line a baking sheet with oven paper. Put 1 cup of the unsweetened shredded coconut on top of the lined baking sheet. Toast in your oven for about 5 minutes making sure that while it toasts to a golden hue, it does not burn.
- Combine the almond flour together with the toasted shredded coconut, the untoasted shredded coconut, the

sweetener, the aquafaba, the almond extract and the salt in a medium sized bowl and blend well.

- Using a tablespoon, scoop out a portion one at a time and form the dough into balls. Place the balls onto the parchment lined baking sheet.
- Bake in the preheated oven for 20 minutes until golden brown in color. Remove from the oven. Set aside and allow them to cool.
- Select a microwave safe bowl and melt the dark chocolate chips. Pick up each macaroon carefully and dip each one singularly into the melted chocolate before returning them to the baking sheet. If there is leftover chocolate, sprinkle it on top of the macaroons and then refrigerate before enjoying.

Vegetarian Keto Chocolate Hazelnut Cookies

Scrumptious no bake Keto cookies that are sugar free and low carb and taste like Ferrero Rocher candies!

- Prep Time: 5 minutes
- Cooking time: 5 minutes
- Yields: Twenty cookies

What you need:

- ¾ cup of coconut flour
- 2 cups of homemade chocolate hazelnut spread *
- ½ cup of sweetener, preferably sticky such as Monk fruit maple syrup
- 1 cup of hazelnuts, crushed
- 1 tablespoon of a liquid of your choosing only if the batter is too thick ù

**For your homemade hazelnut spread, blend together 2lbs. of roasted, skinless roasted hazelnuts, ¾ cup of a sweetener and ½ cup of cocoa powder.*

What to do:

- Line a large baking sheet or dish with parchment paper and set aside.
- In a good-sized bowl, mix all your ingredients well to form a dough. If the batter is too thick, add a little liquid of your choice.

- Place the crushed hazelnuts in a second bowl. Now roll the dough into small balls. Roll each ball in turn in the crushed hazelnuts and then place on the lined plate or baking sheet. Press each ball into a cookie and refrigerate your cookies until firm.
- You can sprinkle them with melted dark chocolate if so desired.

Vegetarian Keto No Bake Chocolate Coconut Crack Bars

A great way to enjoy both chocolate and coconut together, in a sweet but healthy treat for after dinner or snacks.

- Prep Time: 2 minutes
- Cooking time: 5 minutes
- Yields: Twenty cookies

What you need:

- 3 cups of unsweetened shredded coconut flakes
- 1 cup of melted coconut oil
- ¼ cup of Monk fruit maple syrup
- 2 cups of sugar free chocolate chips

What to do:

- Line a pan, which is 8 x 10 inches in size with oven paper and put aside.
- In a good-sized bowl, mix the ingredients well. Now pour the dough into the lined pan and press the dough firmly into place. Put in the refrigerator or into your freezer.
- Once the batter is firm, remove from the refrigerator or freezer and cut into bars. Put the bars back into the refrigerator.
- Melt the chocolate chips of your choice and dip each bar individually in the chocolate. The chocolate should cover the bars in evenly. Refrigerate again until the chocolate is completely firmed up.

Vegetarian Coconut Snowball Cookies

No bake Keto cookies that are low on carbs and huge on taste!

- Prep Time: 5 minutes
- Cooking time: 0 minutes
- Yields: 40 cookies

What you need:

- 4 cups of unsweetened coconut shredded
- extra unsweetened shredded coconut
- 2 tablespoons of granulated erythritol
- ¼ cup of cocoa powder
- 1 cup of chilled coconut cream, not milk

What to do:

- In your blender, combine the shredded coconut, cocoa powder and granulated sweetener and mix on high until well blended.
- Now add the chilled coconut cream and mix until you achieve a thick batter. If necessary, cover and refrigerate until chilled.
- Once chilled, row portions of the batter into small balls. Place the balls on a parchment lined dish or baking sheet. Press each ball into a cookie. Roll your cookie in some extra shredded coconut. Serve and enjoy!

Vegetarian Keto Carrot Cake Bites

Remember Mom's carrot cake? Here's the next best thing. Low carb and sugar-free, these addictive little carrot cakes are perfect for holidays, dessert or snacks.

- Prep Time: 5 minutes
- Cooking time: 0 minutes
- Yields: 15 carrot bites

What you need:

- ½ cup of coconut flour
- ½ cup of water and 1 tablespoon of water
- 2 tablespoons of unsweetened applesauce
- ½ teaspoon of vanilla extract
- 1 teaspoon of cinnamon
- 4 tablespoons of granulated monk fruit sweetener
- 1 shredded medium carrot
- 4 tablespoons of unsweetened shredded coconut

What to do:

- Mix the coconut flour, applesauce, water, and vanilla extract in a bowl and stir, blending well.

- Now add in the monk fruit sweetener, cinnamon and shredded carrot to your mixture. Blend well.
- Refrigerate your batter for 15 to 20 minutes.
- In a separate dish, place your shredded coconut.
- Remove the dough from the refrigerator and roll portions of it into 15 equally sized balls. Now roll the balls in the shredded coconut, coating evenly.
- Keep refrigerated until serving.

Vegetarian Keto Protein Brownies

Craving a chocolaty brownie treat, but don't want to ruin your keto life style? These keto protein brownies are deliciously fudgy treats for dessert or a snack. And they provide you with a good dose of energetic protein as well.

- Prep Time: 10 minutes
- Cooking time: 45 minutes
- Yields: 8 brownies

What you need:

- 1 ½ cups of water
- ½ cup of peanut butter
- 2 scoops of chocolate protein powder (90 grams)
- ¼ cup of granulated sweetener
- 2 tablespoons of coconut flour
- 2 teaspoons of baking powder

What to do:

- Preheat your oven to 350° Fahrenheit and grease your baking pan.
- In a mixing bowl mix the warm water, peanut butter and the granulated sweetener.
- Now add in the chocolate protein powder, coconut flour and the baking powder, mixing well to form your batter.

- Place the batter into your pan, smoothing it out evenly and bake for 45 minutes until a toothpick comes out clean after poking.
- Remove, cool, slice and enjoy.

Made in the USA
Middletown, DE
02 May 2019